AIDS: The Real Cause

AIDS
The Real Cause

Thomas A. Patterson

2014

To

all the independent thinkers

as well as

all the victims of AIDS

AIDS: The Real Cause
First edition, 2014
Second edition, 2015
All rights reserved.

Thomas Patterson, PhD
th.patterson.phd@gmail.com

Contents

Introduction 1

Part I: What is AIDS?

1. Definition of AIDS 4
2. The HIV Explanation 6
3. Alternative Explanations 8
4. The Forgotten Explanation 10

Part II: Evidence

5. Transmission 14
6. Immunology 16
7. Risk Groups 20
8. Symptoms & Treatment 22
9. Summary 24

Part III: Counter-Arguments

10. Antibiotics work 29
11. AIDS is not Syphilis 32
12. Syphilis is not AIDS 36
13. Anti-Viral Drugs Work 38

Part IV: Outlook

14. The Real Cause? 42
15. Implications 44

Appendix

16. Scientific References 48

Introduction

At a press conference on 23 April 1984, it was announced that the probable cause of AIDS had been found: a virus later called human immunodeficiency virus (HIV).

Since then, every child knows that AIDS is caused by HIV.

Wikipedia tells us that "HIV is the causative agent of AIDS".

Researchers hunt HIV, a UN organization distributes test kits for HIV all over the world, AIDS patients receive HIV medication. Every year on World AIDS Day, people are reminded to prevent HIV infection. Even a Nobel prize was awarded.

But is HIV really the cause of AIDS?

Probably not. At any rate, to this day, HIV has never been observed to kill anything or anyone.

Alternative explanation for AIDS have been proposed, but they couldn't fully convince. Something was missing.

From the very beginning, a small group of doctors and researchers has suspected that mankind was once again misled by an old disease known to historians of medicine as "The Great Imitator", caused by a microbe known to clinicians as "the stealth pathogen": syphilis.

At the time, this suspicion couldn't be substantiated, and so it was soon forgotten – almost.

Yet based on modern research, this book will propose that AIDS is indeed caused by syphilis. The Great Imitator has fooled us once more.

Enjoy reading this book!

Part I: What is AIDS?

1 Definition of AIDS

According to the 1993 definition of the US Center for Disease Control and Prevention (CDC), a patient has AIDS if he or she tests positive for the human immune deficiency virus (HIV) and also presents with one of the following: a CD4+ T immune cell count below 200 cells/µL (or a CD4+ T-cell percentage of total lymphocyte immune cells of less than 14%), or the person has one of the defining illnesses [1].

Defining illnesses, which are the main cause of death of AIDS patients, often break out due to the weakened immune system. Examples of the 27 AIDS-defining illnesses as specified by the US CDC include [2]:

- recurrent pneumonia (an inflammation of the lung alveoli),
- lymphoma (a tumor of lymphoid immune cells),
- Kaposi's Sarcoma (a skin tumor),
- tuberculosis,
- and several other bacterial, fungal and viral infections .

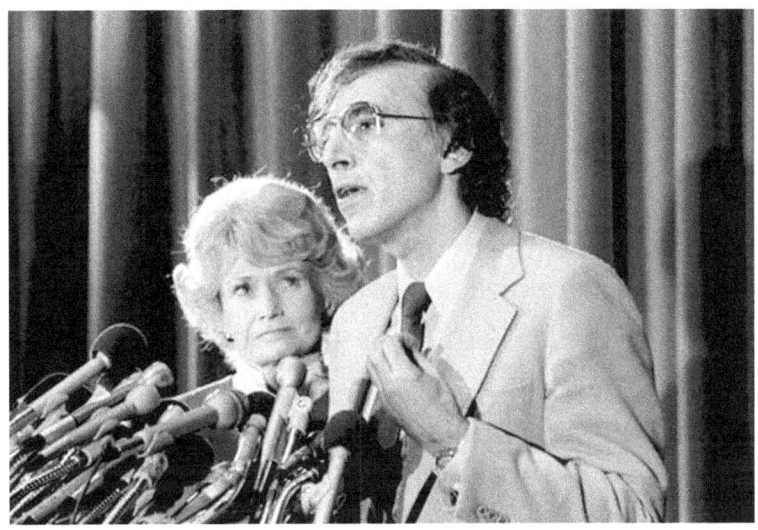

Figure 1: April 23, 1984 – "The probable cause of AIDS has been found." Press conference with Robert Gallo, co-discoverer of the putative HI virus.

2 The HIV Explanation

In search of the cause of AIDS, the lymph node tissues of individuals at risk of AIDS were analyzed during the early 1980s. It was determined that a virus later called human immuodeficiency virus (HIV) is the causal agent of AIDS [3-5].

Since then, several studies have confirmed strong correlations between HIV positivity (i.e., a positive test for HIV) and the development of AIDS, both at the individual and epidemiological levels [6,7]. Moreover, it has been shown that HIV positivity can be transmitted in several ways, including sexual intercourse, infected blood, and *in utero* from an infected mother to her unborn child [8-10].

However, to date no causal mechanism has been found by which the putative HI virus causes the loss of CD4+ T-cells and triggers the onset of AIDS, and *in vitro* and animal experiments have consistently failed to reproduce immunological or clinical symptoms [11-13].

Rather, it has been shown that only 0.00001 to 0.01% of HIV virions are infectious *in vitro* and *in vivo* [14], and more than 95% of dying immune cells are not productively infected but instead correspond to HIV-negative bystander cells [14,15]. In addition, morphologically indistinguishable viral particles were found in activated lymph nodes of HIV-negative individuals [16].

In sum, 30 years after the HIV explanation for AIDS was first proposed, causal evidence is still lacking, fundamental questions remain unanswered, contradictions unresolved, and a vaccine against the putative HI virus is not in sight [17].

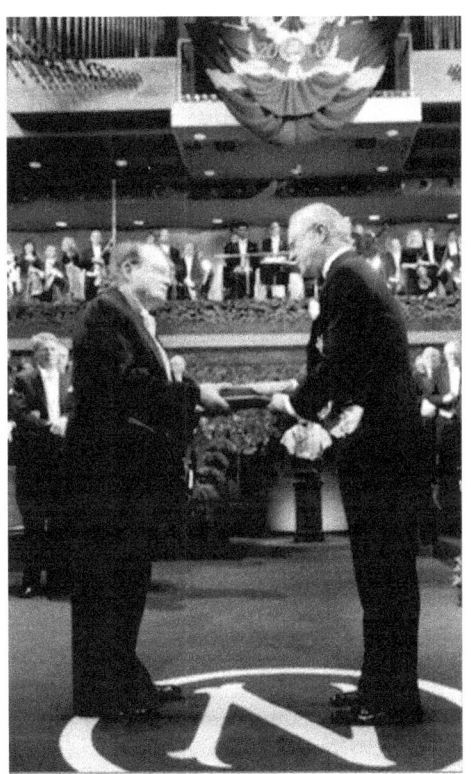

Figure 2: December 7, 2008 – Luc Montagnier receiving the Nobel prize for the co-discovery of the putative HI virus.

3 Alternative Explanations

In view of these shortcomings of the "official" HIV-AIDS hypothesis, some researchers have proposed that AIDS may be caused not by a virus, but instead by the use of narcotics (especially in risk groups in industrial countries) or malnutrition (especially in affected populations in developing countries) [18].

According to this proposal, HIV could be a (harmless) passenger virus [19], or it could not be an exogenous virus at all [20].

However, it remains unclear how conditions such as malnutrition or use of narcotics, while clearly adverse to the immune system in general, may induce the consistent, irreversible loss of CD4+ T-cells observed in AIDS.

Moreover, the correlations between HIV positivity and the onset of AIDS-defining illnesses as well as the observed transmission of HIV positivity have not been convincingly explained by this hypothesis.

Despite these limitations, the alternative explanations have highlighted important aspects that have to be accommodated by any complete explanation of AIDS.

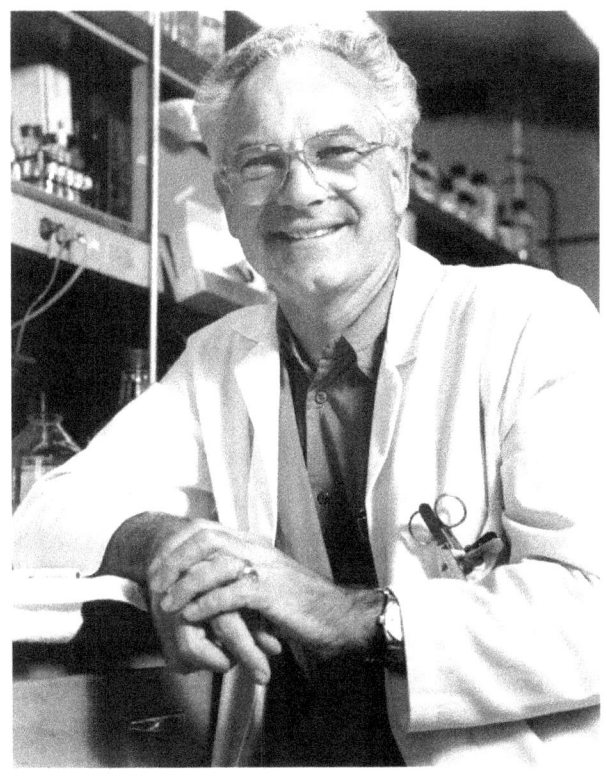

Figure 3: Peter Duesberg, one of the early critics of the HIV explanation, and proponent of the narcotics explanation of AIDS.

4 The Forgotten Explanation

From the very beginning, a small group of doctors and researchers has proposed a third, almost forgotten explanation: AIDS is caused by an infection with spirochete bacteria, notably by Treponema pallidum, the microbe causing syphilis [21-25].

According to this explanation, the onset of AIDS symptoms is triggered by an initial weakening of the immune system, either by the spirochete bacteria themselves, or by external factors, such as drug abuse, poor hygiene, chronic malnutrition, additional infections, severe stress, or improper medication.

In response to this initial perturbation of the immune system, the spirochete bacteria gain the upper hand and attack host organs, including the central nervous system, skin tissues, and key parts of the immune system, notably lymph nodes, thymus and bone marrow.

In turn, this leads to a rapid and persistent deterioration of host immunity and sets the stage for the outbreak of AIDS-defining illnesses. HIV positivity may be seen a marker of this process.

In the next section, the supporting evidence for this explanation will be reviewed. Thereafter, counter-arguments are addressed.

AIDS: The Real Cause

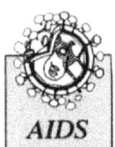
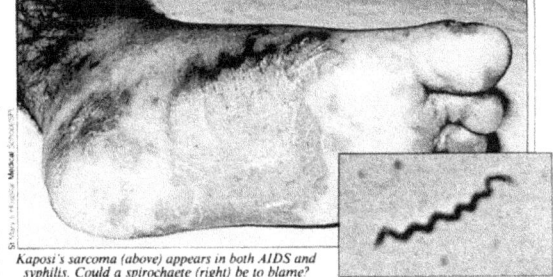

Figure 4: 1987 New Scientist article on the possible link between syphilis and AIDS.

Part II: Evidence

5 Transmission

T. pallidum is transmitted in precisely the same way as HIV positivity: by sexual intercourse, infected blood, and from an infected mother to her newborn child [26,27].

During sexual intercourse, the receiving partner is at a much higher risk of acquiring HIV positivity [28]. The same applies to infections with T. pallidum, especially in men who have sex with men (MSM) [29].

Therefore, the Syphilis-as-AIDS hypothesis fully explains the transmission of HIV positivity and AIDS.

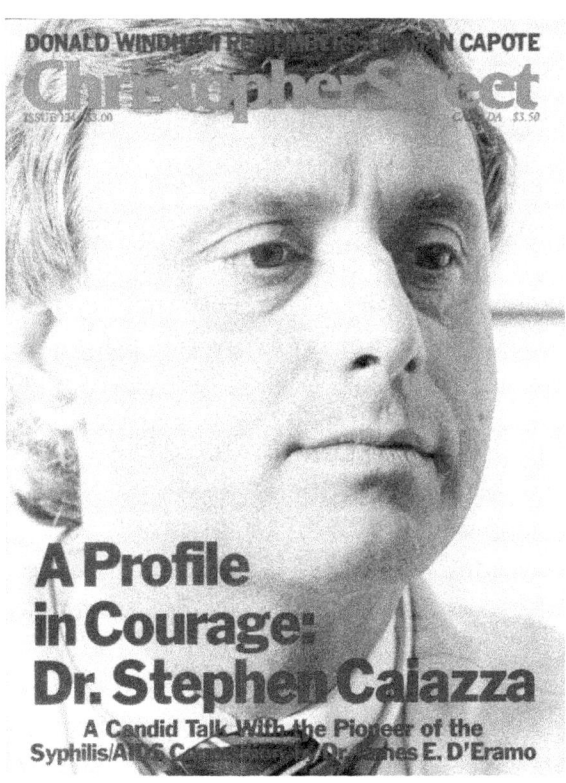

Figure 5: Stephen Caiazza, New York physician and one of the early proponents of the syphilis explanation of AIDS.

6 Immunology

T. pallidum has been shown to invade and kill animal and human B and T immune cells, notably CD4+ T-cells (see Figure 7) [30-34]. Thus, the Syphilis-as-AIDS hypothesis provides a specific causal mechanism by which T. pallidum induces the AIDS-defining depletion of CD4+ T-cells.

T. pallidum and other spirochetes have been shown to invade the human immune system, including thymus and bone marrow, where they may interfere with and prevent the formation of CD4+ T-cells (see Figure 9) [35-37]. This would explain why the transplantation of bone marrow has a beneficial effect on the course of AIDS [38].

T. pallidum and other spirochetes have been shown to induce the expression of precisely the same T-cell coreceptors as implicated in the transmission and replication of the putative HI virus: CCR5 and CXCR4 [39-42]. Therefore, the Syphilis-as-AIDS hypothesis naturally explains the observed expression of these coreceptors in AIDS patients. Indeed, spirochetes and/or spirochetal products have the capacity to bring together all of the cellular elements and surface molecules observed during a putative HIV infection [43].

One of the strongest predictors of disease progression in AIDS is T-cell activation. The frequency of circulating cells that express surface receptors CD38 and HLA-DR (which are markers of cell activation) predict the rate of CD4+ T-cell decline. This effect appears to be independent of putative viral load [44]. Strikingly, the specific T-cell receptor pattern observed in syphilis, especially late-stage syphilis, is identical [41].

An existing infection with T. pallidum facilitates the transmission of HIV positivity [45,46]. This is predicted by the Syphilis-as-AIDS hypothesis.

An existing infection with T. pallidum is associated with a higher so-called viral load, and a lower CD4+ T-cell count in HIV positive patients [48,49]. This is predicted by the Syphilis-as-AIDS hypothesis.

Monkeys infected with T. pallidum developed anorexia and died of Pneumocystis carinii, an AIDS-defining illness, after 44 months [50]. This is precisely what is observed in AIDS patients. Thus, the Syphilis-as-AIDS hypothesis causally explains how AIDS patients lose their CD4+ T-cells and become susceptible to AIDS-defining illnesses.

T. pallidum is able to induce every antigen/antibody band considered indicative of a putative HIV infection in standard test methods (i.e., p17, p24, p41, gp120/160) [51-54]. In other words, a syphilis infection by itself may cause an HIV positive test result. Indeed, experiments have shown that rabbits infected with putative HIV became HIV positive only after super-infection with syphilis [55].

T. pallidum induces the expression of putative HIV genes in human immune cells [56]. In rabbits, HIV gene expression was detectable *only* after super-infection with T. pallidum [55]. In *in vitro* experiments, human T-cells release viral-like particles not spontaneously, but only after intensive immunogenic stimulation [57]

In 2007, researchers using PCR found that intestinal bacteria of AIDS patients are bearing genetic sequences for more than 90% identical with those of HIV-1 [47].

T. pallidum has a highly reduced genome and is unable to live outside its human host. It has been shown that T. pallidum and other spirochetes employ viral-like particles and reverse transcriptase activity to interact with host cells [58-60]. This could explain the detection of reverse transcriptase and other viral aspects by HIV test methods.

In sum, the Syphilis-as-AIDS hypothesis explains all of the immunological and clinical aspects of HIV positivity and AIDS.

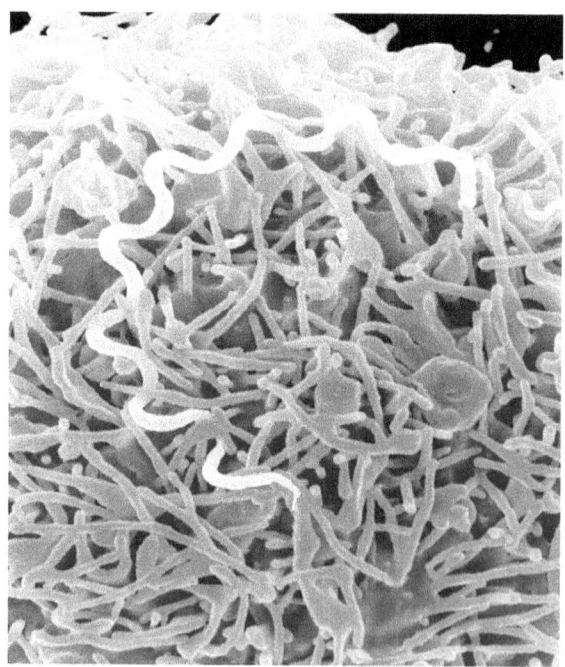

Figure 6: Treponema pallidum on the surface of a human immune cell [100].

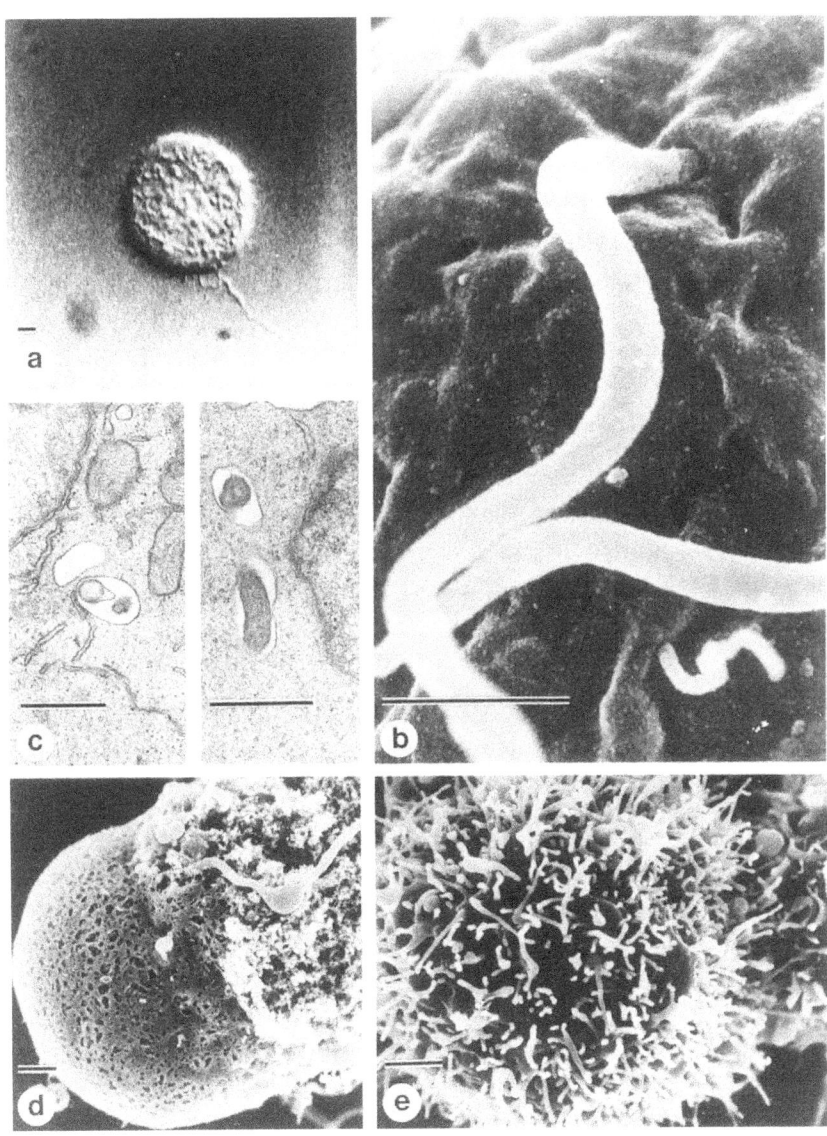

Figure 7: T. pallidum entering and destroying a human immune cell [30].

7 Risk Groups

Both the prevalence and incidence of HIV positivity have been shown to correlate strongly with acute or prior syphilis infection [22-25,27,61-63]. This is predicted by the Syphilis-as-AIDS hypothesis.

The global prevalence of syphilis matches perfectly with the prevalence of the putative HI virus. It is highest in MSM of industrial countries as well as in the population of several developing regions, notably sub-Saharan Africa [25,62]. A country that is particularly affected by AIDS is also highly exposed to syphilis: South Africa [64].

Patients testing positive for HIV, especially MSM, have a very high prevalence of intestinal spirochetosis (see Figure 8) [65-67].

In parts of Africa, the prevalence of intestinal spirochetosis is close to one hundred percent, affecting both men and women [68].

For heterosexual women in developed countries, anal intercourse is by far the most risky sexual practice to acquire HIV positivity or AIDS [73].

The high prevalence of intestinal spirochetosis is especially relevant, given that the gut-associated lymphoid tissue (GALT) plays a key role in the onset and progression of AIDS [127].

Therefore, the Syphilis-as-AIDS hypothesis perfectly explains the observed pattern of AIDS risk groups, both in developed and in developing countries.

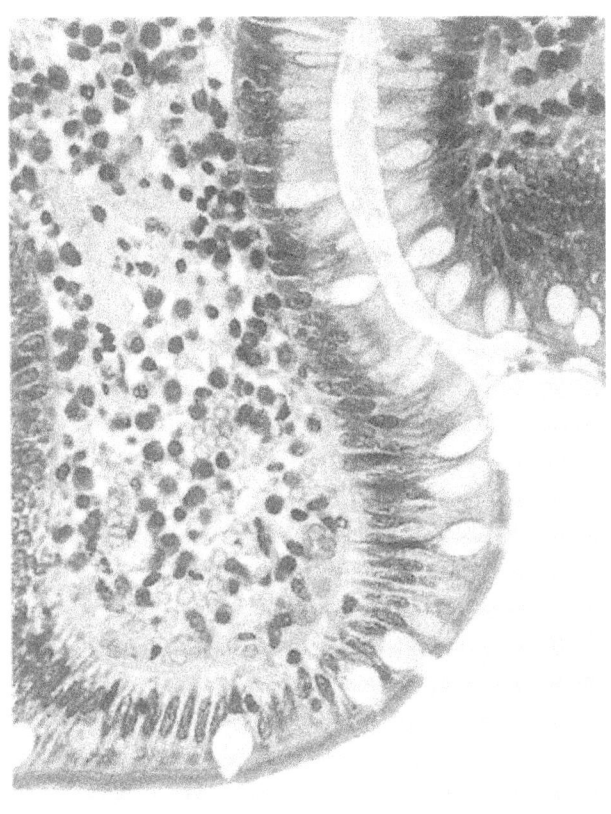

Figure 8: Intestinal spirochetosis (border on the edge of the colonic epithelium, lower half of the image) [65].

8 Symptoms & Treatment

Spirochetes have been shown to induce severe local oxidative stress to host cells [69]. This could potentially lead to mitochondrial dysfunction and the onset of tumors such as the AIDS-defining Kaposi's Sarcoma [70]. Additional factors causing oxidative stress, such as drug abuse or chronic malnutrition, could significantly contribute to this effect.

Spirochetes proliferate fastest at temperatures somewhat below 37 degrees Celsius [26], which is why the skin may be heavily affected syphilis and other spirochete infections [27]. According to the Syphilis-as-AIDS hypothesis, this would also explain why the skin of many AIDS patients is affected by the disease.

During the 1980s, doctors who, instead of prescribing anti-retroviral drugs, applied a classic syphilis treatment to AIDS patients, i.e., antibiotics, reported not only a massive drop in mortality, but also a reversal of Kaposi's Sarcoma [24]. In fact, Kaposi's Sarcoma was successfully treated with Penicillin already as of the 1950s [71,72].

Prior to the classification as AIDS, each and every of the AIDS-defining illnesses had already been associated with syphilis for decades, if not centuries (since the first unambiguous description of syphilis at the end of the fifteenth century) [74,75]. This includes hallmark conditions such as Kaposi's Sarcoma [24,76] (which was first described by Moritz Kaposi in 1872 in the Journal of Syphilology and Dermatology [77]), as well as lymphadentopathy (enlarged lymph nodes) [78] and lymphoma (tumerous lymph nodes) [79-82] and all of the secondary infections, including notably tuberculosis [83,84].

To date, the 30 year quest for developing an HIV vaccine has failed [13,57]. This is predicted by the Syphilis-as-AIDS hypothesis.

Therefore, the Syphilis-as-AIDS hypothesis fully explains the observed symptoms of AIDS, the successful treatment of Kaposi's Sarcoma by penicillin, and the failed search for a vaccine.

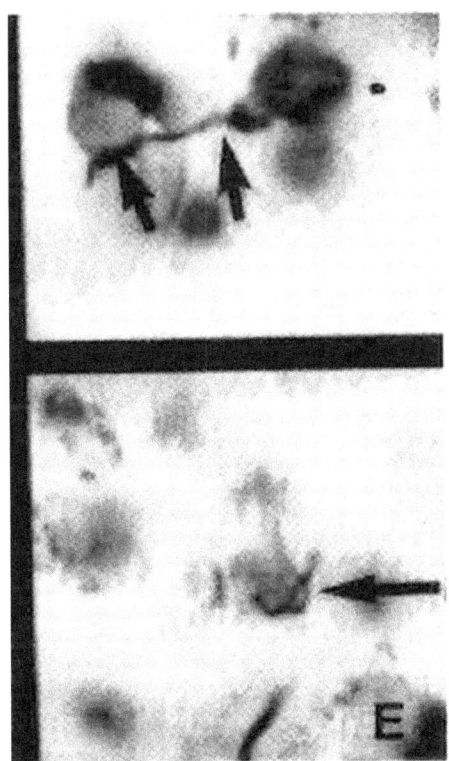

Figure 9: Spirochetes in human bone marrow [36].

9 Summary

In sum, the Syphilis-as-AIDS hypothesis appears to comprehensively and causally explain AIDS, including its immunological, clinical and epidemiological aspects as well as its correlation with HIV positivity.

Furthermore, it agrees with the observation that additional oxidative stress, induced by drug abuse, chronic malnutrition, or other sources, may significantly exacerbate the course of a syphilis infection and trigger the onset of AIDS.

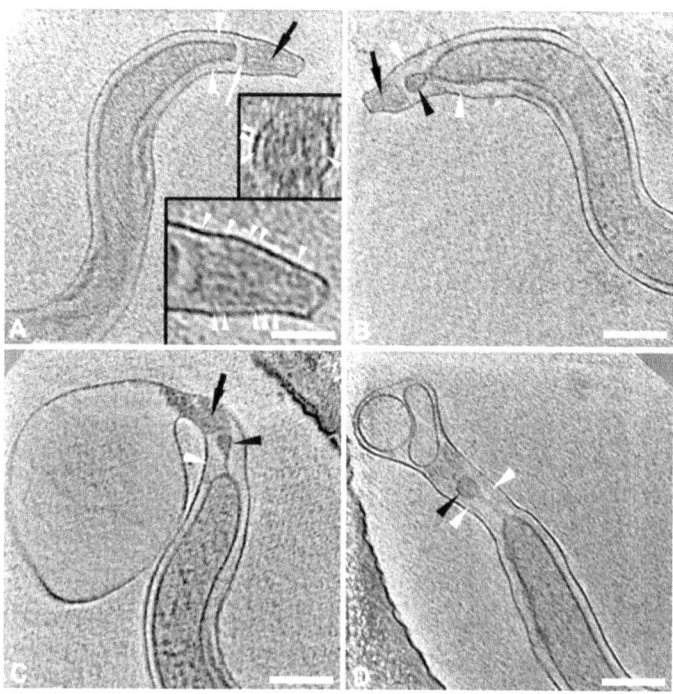

Figure 10: Details of T. pallidum architecture. [Izard, 2009]

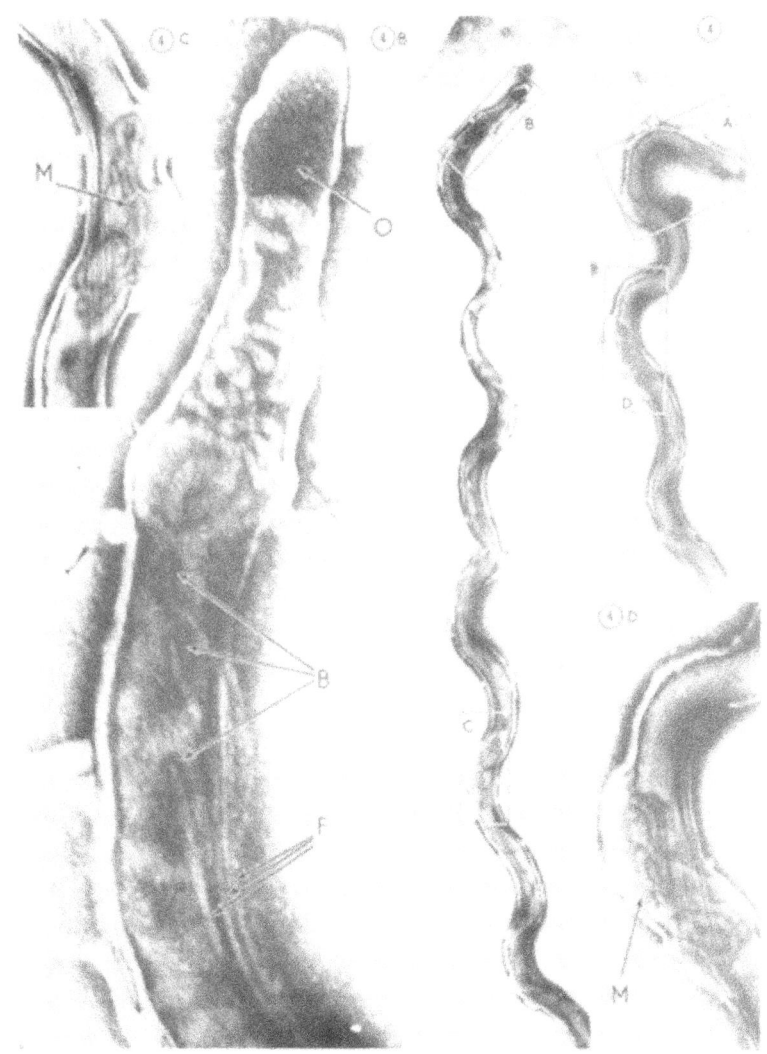

Figure 11: T. pallidum morphology. [98]

Part III: Counter-Arguments

10 Antibiotics work

Counter-argument: Syphilis and other spirochete infections are treated and cured with antibiotics. Therefore, spirochetes cannot be the cause of AIDS.

Standard antibiotics may be able to suppress acute symptoms of spirochete infections such as syphilis or Lyme disease, but they have repeatedly failed to eliminate the actual infection [22-25,74,85-91]. This is for several reasons. Within hours of an infection, spirochete bacteria can invade the central nervous system (see Figure 13) [92], where they are protected from the reach of several standard antibiotics that cannot cross the blood-brain-barrier. Specifically, it has been pointed out that the standard antibiotic used to treat syphilis in the U.S. and elsewhere during the forty years prior to the AIDS epidemic, benzathine penicillin, cannot cross the blood-brain-barrier [24, 93, 94].

Also, spirochetes can easily penetrate host cells – even host immune cells – and continue proliferating inside cells, shielded from the effect of many standard antibiotics (see Figure 15 [95-97].

Finally, if exposed to conditions adverse to growth – such as antibiotics or a shortage of nutrients – spirochetes form so-called cysts or round-bodies (see Figure 12). This metabolically inactive form allows spirochetes to evade and survive adverse conditions for months, years, or even decades, before reactivating their metabolism and resuming growth and proliferation, as has been repeatedly observed, both *in vitro* and *in vivo* [59,60,74,87,98,99].

Thus, it is likely that substantial reservoirs of latent T. pallidum infections persisted even in treated patients, especially among risk groups such as MSM, prior to the outbreak of the AIDS epidemic [22,24]. Already in the 1960s and 1970s, syphilis researchers observed that "under the influence of biological conditions unknown to us, these treponemes may regain all or part of their virulence and become pathogenic, at any rate in regard to their host. When treatment is started late, a curious state of equilibrium has been created between the host, mobilizing his defences, and the parasite occurring in the tissues. This latent condition, like 'clinical cure', by no means indicates bacteriological sterilization." (see Figure 14) [87]

It was also known that immunosuppressive drugs, such as cortisone, may reactivate latent syphilis [85]. It is reasonable to expect that abuse of recreational and prescribed drugs by risk groups such as MSM during the 1970s and 1980s had the same effect [22]. It is noteworthy that the activation of latent syphilis in HIV-infected individuals appears to coincide with the development of immune depression [27,100].

Therefore, rather than refuting the Syphilis-as-AIDS hypothesis, these observations may actually explain the peculiar progression and the long incubation periods of AIDS, as well as its interdependence with external factors.

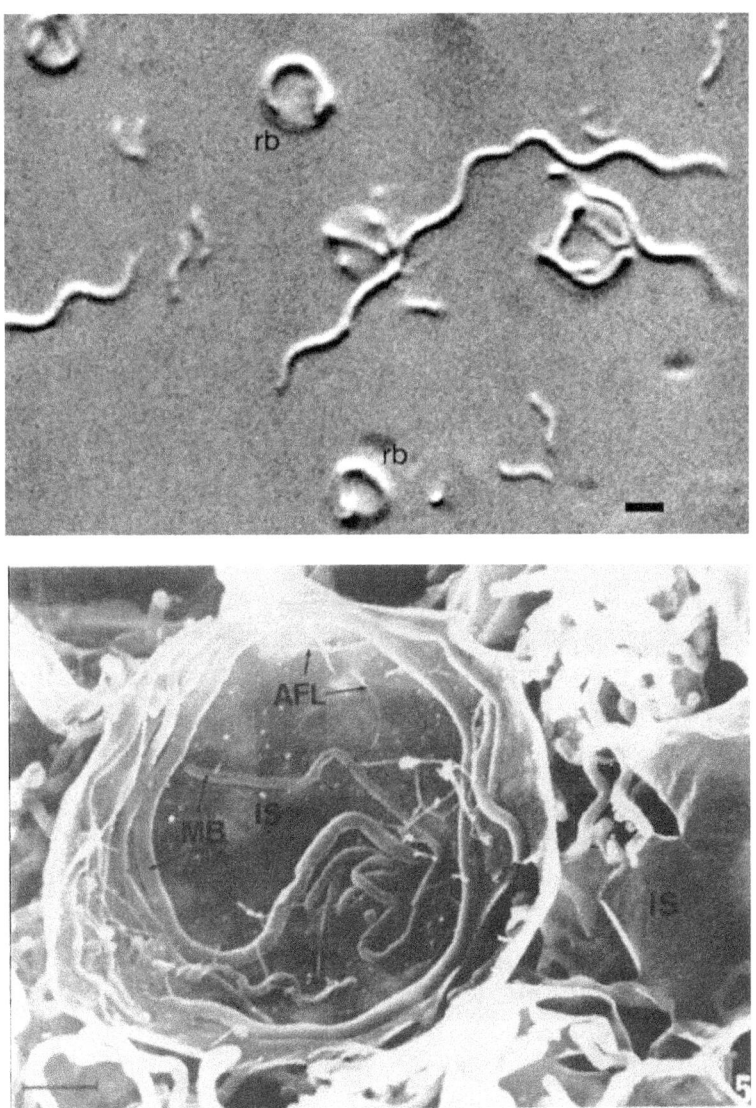

Figure 12: Spirochete round bodies (cysts). [60,99]

11 AIDS is not Syphilis

Counter-argument: Not every AIDS patient has syphilis, or is infected with spirochetes.

In the 1980s, it was estimated that more than 60% of the (urban) gay community had a history of syphilis and 90% of those with AIDS had had one or more syphilitic infections [22,27]. In parts of sub-Saharan Africa, it is estimated that up to 80% of the population are infected with syphilis, often as of birth [25,62-64]. Given the arguments above concerning the ability of T. pallidum to evade antibiotic treatments, it is reasonable to assume that many syphilis infections have in fact never been truly cured and continue to persist in a chronic or latent state.

Nevertheless, there remains a number of AIDS cases that do not test positive for syphilis, and may not even have a history of syphilitic infections. This seems to contradict the Syphilis-as-AIDS hypothesis. However, it is well known that current syphilis test methods are prone to false-negative results, i.e., they do not detect an existing infection [101-107]. This is for several reasons. First of all, most test methods rely on the host immune response to antigens specific or non-specific to T. pallidum (i.e., treponemal and non-treponemal test). However, T. pallidum is exceedingly good in evading a host immune response and achieving kind of a symbiotic relationship with host cells [53,108].

This is because T. pallidum features an outer membrane that is extremely sparse in antigenic proteins [109-113]. Moreover, in case of an immune response, T. pallidum can change these antigens by adapting gene expression [114,115].

On top of that, the weaker the immune system, the less likely it is to respond to the presence and activity of spirochetes [22,33,74]. This is exactly what has been observed in HIV/AIDS patients: Reactivity of syphilis tests decreases significantly as the disease progresses [74,101-107]. Syphilis itself is known to induce an immune-suppressive effect, especially in its late stages [116,117]. Additional sources of oxidative stress, such as drug abuse or chronic malnutrition, further weaken the immune response and thus raise the probability of false-negative test results [22].

Apparently, the lowest sensitivity is achieved by using a non-treponemal test (e.g., a *venereal disease research laboratory (VDRL)* test or a *rapid plasma reagin (RPR)* test) as a screening test and thereafter a treponemal test (e.g., a *fluorescent treponemal antibody absorption (FTA-ABS)* test or a *treponema pallidum particle agglutination assay (TPPA)* test) as confirmatory test. The sensitivity of this procedure may be as low as 20% [24,74]. This test method is, however, the standard procedure in most parts of the world, including the U.S. and Europe [74, 118]. In other words, actual syphilis infections, especially in risk groups, may be up to five times more common than previously thought.

In addition, it turns out that even the detection of T. pallidum gene fragments in blood serum by PCR has a sensitivity of as low as 24% [119,120]. To date, it appears that the only test methods with a reasonably high sensitivity, even in immunosuppressed patients, are the direct inspection of (potentially) infected tissues by PCR or dark-field microscopy [74,118,119].

It is interesting to note that in the middle of 19th century, it was discovered that repeated infection with T. pallidum leads to an apparent cure of syphilis: symptoms disappear and remain absent even after re-infection [74,121,122]. In the false belief of inducing some sort of immunity, this led some doctors to administer several doses of T. pallidum to their syphilis patients, a controversial procedure called syphilization, which was abandoned only towards the end of the 19th century [123]. It seems quite likely, however, that risk groups such as MSM inadvertently exposed themselves to a large-scale syphilization experiment during the decades prior to the AIDS epidemic, an experiment further complicated by the repeated use of illicit drugs and unsuitable medication.

In sum, this means that a large number of patients infected with syphilis may have been missed so far. Also, the fact that AIDS patients often do not test positive for syphilis is not in contradiction, but rather to be expected according to the Syphilis-as-AIDS hypothesis, given that their immunological response is severely impaired. Therefore, based on current standard test methods, this counter-argument does not refute the Syphilis-as-AIDS hypothesis.

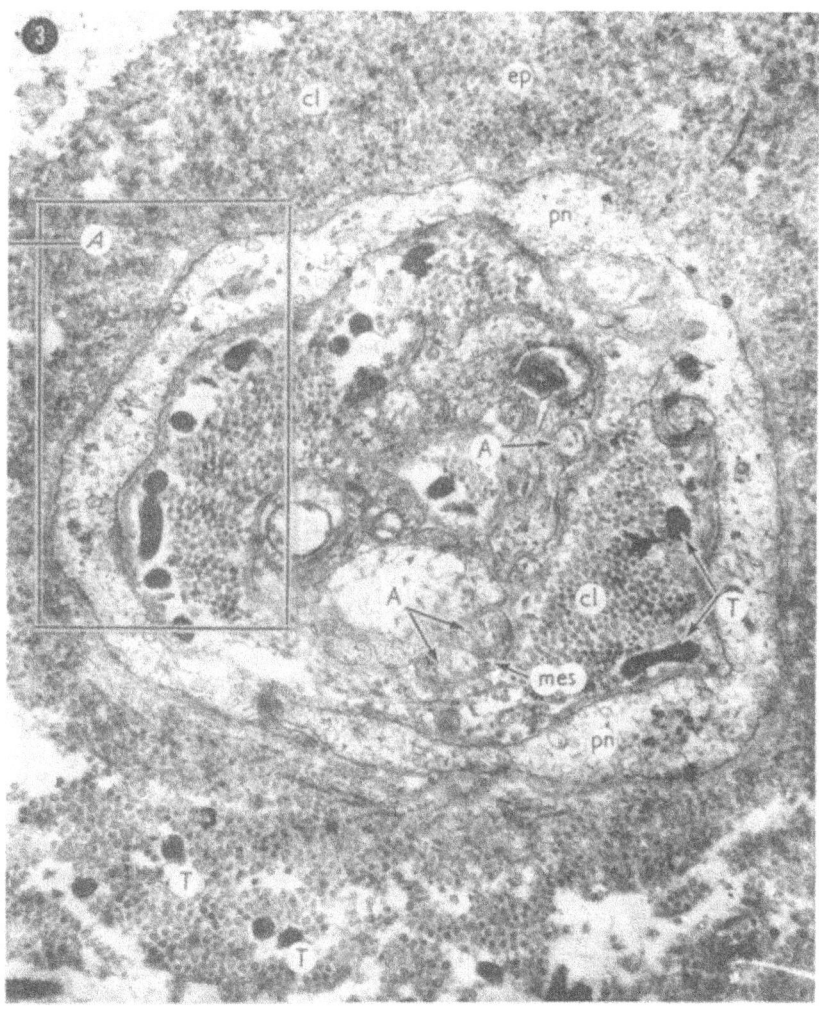

Figure 13: T. pallidum (dark structures) inside rabbit nerve fibers. [92]

12 Syphilis is not AIDS

Counter-argument: Not every patient infected with syphilis develops AIDS.

This is correct. However, not every person infected with T. pallidum develops late-stage syphilis [100]. Also, not every patient infected with the putative HI virus has developed AIDS [124].

While the Syphilis-as-AIDS hypothesis proposes that AIDS is caused by T. pallidum, this does not imply that every infection with T. pallidum leads to HIV positivity, or AIDS. It is likely that the progression of an infection with T. pallidum to late-stage syphilis, or AIDS, is influenced by several factors, including the amount and strains of spirochetes, as well as the strength of the patient's immune system. The latter aspect is in line with the observed effects of drug abuse and malnutrition on the progression of AIDS.

Therefore, this counter-argument, while true, does not refute the Syphilis-as-AIDS hypothesis. Rather, it shows that additional factors causing oxidative stress and immuno-suppression are often required to turn a normal syphilis infection into malignant syphilis, which may then be diagnosed as AIDS.

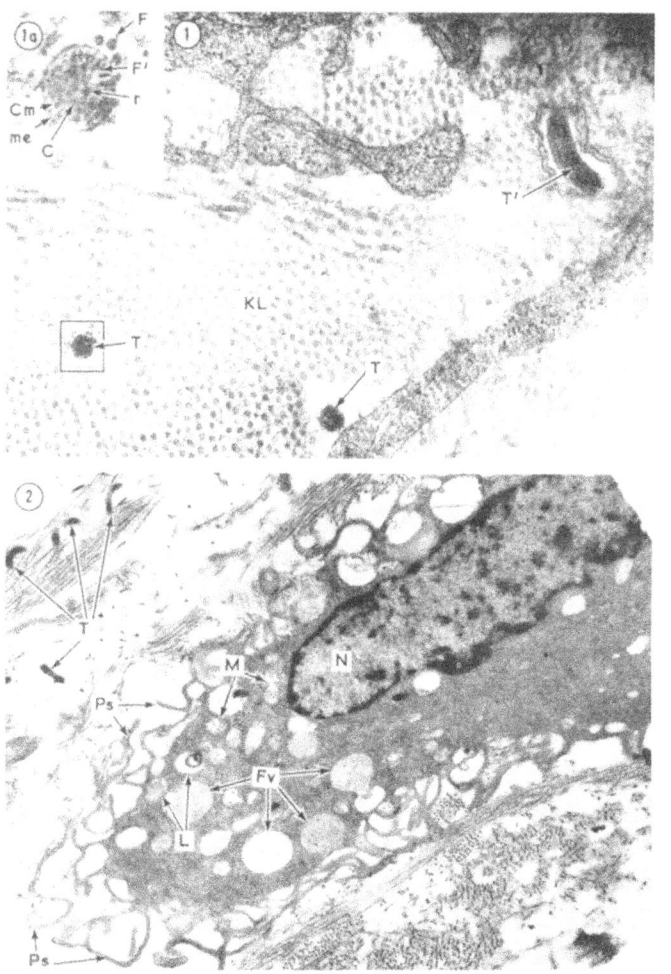

Figure 14: Viable T. pallidum in a rabbit after treatment with penicillin.[86]

13 Anti-Viral Drugs Work

Counter-argument: Highly active anti-retroviral therapy (HAART) has been shown to be effective against AIDS.

Indeed, HAART has been shown to ameliorate or retard the onset and progression of AIDS and its defining illnesses.

However, besides its anti-retroviral effects, HAART has general antibiotic effects. Specifically, HAART is known to be partially effective against syphilis [125]. According to the Syphilis-as-AIDS hypothesis, this could in fact explain why HAART is partially effective against AIDS. In turn, it was shown that treatment of AIDS-related co-infections lowers so-called viral load [126].

Thus, this counter-argument does not refute the Syphilis-as-AIDS hypothesis. Rather, it is in line with its predictions.

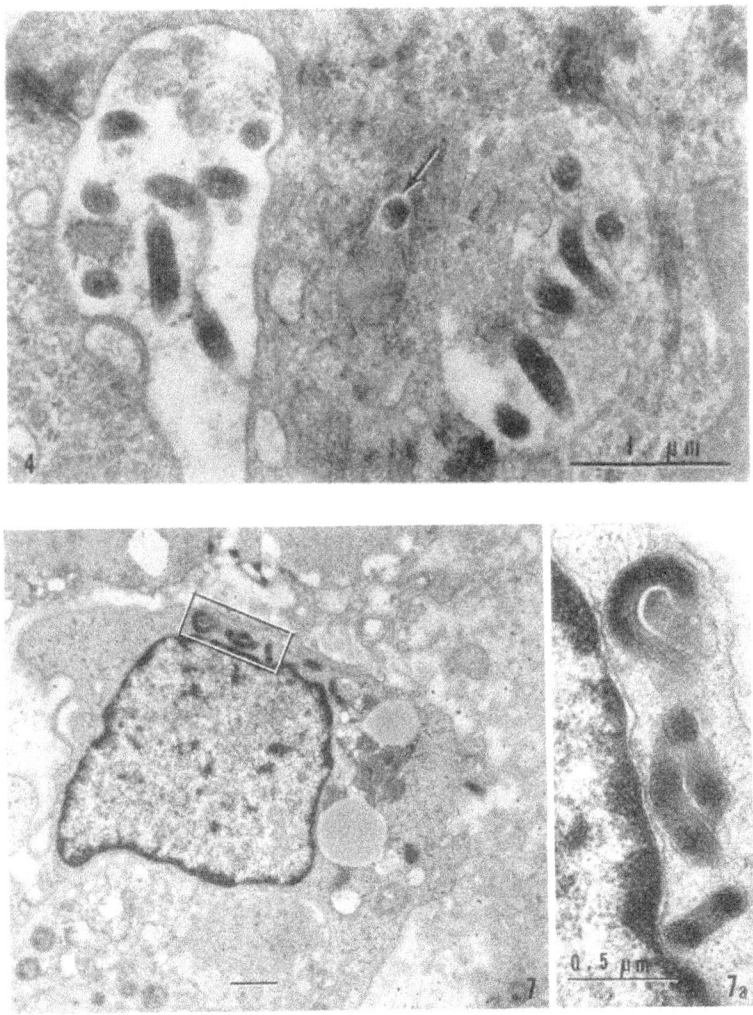

Figure 15: T. pallidum inside rabbit cells. [95, 96]

Part IV: Outlook

14 The Real Cause?

To verify or falsify the hypothesis that AIDS is caused by syphilis, the following experiments are proposed:

1. Testing of AIDS patients for T. pallidum, using direct observational methods such as dark-field microscopy, antigen testing, and PCR.

2. Examining the tissues of patients that have died from AIDS for spirochetes, especially in parts of the body related to the immune system, such as bone marrow, lymph nodes, thymus, and spleen.

3. Testing the impact of syphilis treatment on key indicators of AIDS, including viral load, CD4+ T-cell count, and progression of AIDS-defining illnesses. Of particular interest would be the use of advanced antibiotics that reach the central nervous system and are effective intra-cellularly and against inactive spirochete round-bodies. Such a treatment should be most effective not only against syphilis, but also against AIDS.

4. Testing, in vitro or in animals, whether HIV positivity can be induced by infection with T. pallidum.

5. Testing whether AIDS-like symptoms can be induced in animals by infecting them, repeatedly, with spirochete bacteria.

The Syphilis-as-AIDS hypothesis is refuted, at least partially, if T. pallidum cannot be detected, with state-of-the-art methods, in each and every AIDS patient (as defined by the CDC 1993 classification), unless the patient turns out to be false-positive regarding HIV and has accidentally acquired an AIDS-defining illness due to another reason.

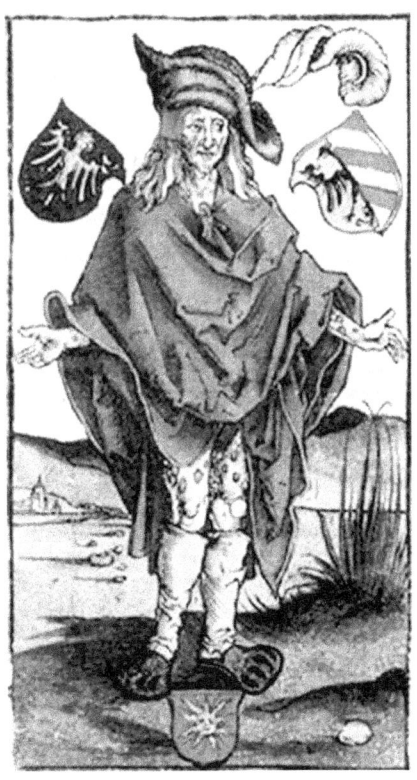

Figure 16: A Syphilitic Man (Albrecht Duerer, 1496)

15 Implications

If the Syphilis-as-AIDS hypothesis turns out to be correct, it is suggested to focus AIDS therapy on the development of antibiotics or other forms of treatment that are highly effective against spirochetes such as T. pallidum, as well as to further improve testing methods for spirochete infections, and to raise public awareness regarding the risk and prevention of an infection with spirochetes.

The Syphilis-as-AIDS hypothesis implies that as of the 1980s, existing syphilis-related diseases have been reclassified as AIDS in the presence of a positive result of the newly developed and introduced HIV test.

If so, HIV positivity has been an epidemic of a new test method, not an epidemic of a virus. AIDS has been a new edition of an old disease: syphilis.

> *"Know syphilis in all its manifestations and relations, and all other things clinical will be added unto you."*
>
> *Sir William Osler, 1897*

Appendix

16 Scientific References

1. US Center for Disease Control and Prevention. 1993 Revised Classification System for HIV Infection and Expanded Surveillance Case Definition for AIDS Among Adolescents and Adults. Published on December 18, 1992. Online at http://www.cdc.gov/mmwr/preview/mmwrhtml/00018871.htm, accessed on December 18, 2013.

2. US Center for Disease Control and Prevention. AIDS-Defining Conditions. Published on December 18, 1992. Online at http://www.cdc.gov/mmwr/preview/mmwrhtml/rr5710a2.htm, accessed on December 18, 2013.

3. Barré-Sinoussi F, Chermann JC, Rey F, et al. Isolation of a T-lymphotropic retrovirus from a patient at risk for acquired immune deficiency syndrome (AIDS). *Science* 1983; 220 (4599): 868–71.

4. Popovic M, Sarngadharan MG, Read E, Gallo RC. Detection, isolation, and continuous production of cytopathic retroviruses (HTLV-III) from patients with AIDS and pre-AIDS. *Science* 1984; 224 (4648): 497–500.

5. Gallo RC, Montagnier L. The chronology of AIDS research. *Nature* 1987; 326 (6112): 435–6.

6. Pantaleo G, Graziosi C, Fauci AS. New concepts in the immunopathogenesis of human immunodeficiency virus infection. *N Engl J Med.* 1993; 328 (5): 327–35.

7. Douek DC, Picker LJ, Koup RA. T cell dynamics in HIV-1 infection. *Annu Rev Immunol.* 2003; 21: 265–304.

8. Connor RI, Ho DD. Transmission and pathogenesis of human immunodeficiency virus type 1. *AIDS Res Hum Retroviruses* 1994;10 (4): 321–3.

9. Goedert JJ, Kessler CM, Aledort LM, et al. A prospective study of human immunodeficiency virus type 1 infection and the development of AIDS in subjects with hemophilia. *N Engl J Med* 1989; 321 (17): 1141–8.

10. European Collaborative Study. Risk factors for mother-to-child transmission of HIV-1. *Lancet* 1992; 339: 1007–12.

11   Gorry PR, Churchill M, Crowe SM, Cunningham AL, Gabuzda D. Pathogenesis of macrophage tropic HIV-1. *Curr HIV Res.* 2005; 3 (1): 53–60.

12   Glushakova S, Grivel JC, Fitzgerald W, Sylwester A, Zimmerberg J, Margolis LB. Evidence for the HIV-1 phenotype switch as a causal factor in acquired immunodeficiency. *Nat Med.* 1998; 4 (3): 346–9.

13   Mishra S, Dwivedi SP, Dwivedi N, Singh RB. Immune Response and Possible Causes of CD4+T-cell Depletion in Human Immunodeficiency Virus (HIV) - 1 Infection. The Open Nutraceuticals Journal 2009; 2: 46-51.

14   Février M, Dorgham K, Rebollo A. CD4+ T Cell Depletion in Human Immunodeficiency Virus (HIV) Infection: Role of Apoptosis. Viruses. 2011 May; 3(5): 586–612.

15   Doitsh G, Cavrois M, Lassen KG, et al. Abortive HIV infection mediates CD4 T cell depletion and inflammation in human lymphoid tissue. Cell. 2010 Nov 24;143(5):789-801.

16   O'Hara CJ, Groopman JE, Federman M. The ultrastructural and immunohistochemical demonstration of viral particles in lymph nodes from human immunodeficiency virus-related and non-human immunodeficiency virus-related lymphadenopathy syndromes. Hum Pathol. 1988 May;19(5):545-9.

17   Cummins NW, Badley AD. Anti-apoptotic mechanisms of HIV: lessons and novel approaches to curing HIV. Cell Mol Life Sci. 2013; 70: 3355–3363.

18   Duesberg PH. AIDS acquired by drug consumption and other noncontagious risk factors. *Pharmacol Ther* 1992; 55 (3): 201–77.

19   Duesberg PH, Mandrioli D, McCormack A, et al. AIDS since 1984: No evidence for a new, viral epidemic – not even in Africa. *Ital J Anat Embryol.* 2011; 116(2): 73–92.

20   Papadopulos-Eleopulos E, Turner VF, Papadimitriou J, et al. A critique of the Montagnier evidence for the HIV/AIDS hypothesis. *Med Hypotheses.* 2004; 63(4): 597–601.

21 Dierig KU, Waldthaler U. Immundefekt - ein Vorstadium? Selecta 1985; 36: 3231-3235

22 McKenna J. "Unmasking AIDS: Chemical Immunosuppression and Seronegative Syphilis," Medical Hypothesis, vol. 21 (1986): 425.

23 Coulter H. AIDS and Syphilis: The Hidden Link. North Atlantic Books, USA.

24 Caiazza S. Chronic Spirochetal Infection and the Pathogenesis of AIDS. Quantum Medicine 1988; 1(1): 117-27.

25 Mitchell RB. Syphilis as AIDS?--A call for research. Med Hypotheses. 1993 Aug;41(2):115-7.

26 Porcella SF, Schwan TG. Borrelia burgdorferi and Treponema pallidum: a comparison of functional genomics, environmental adaptations, and pathogenic mechanisms. *J Clin Invest.* 2001; 107 (6): 651–656.

27 Zetola NM, Klausner JD. Syphilis and HIV Infection: An Update. Clin Infect Dis. 2007 May 1;44(9):1222-8.

28 Padian NS, Shiboski SC, Jewell NP. Female-to-male transmission of human immunodeficiency virus. JAMA. 1991 Sep 25;266(12):1664-7.

29 Whitlow CB. Bacterial Sexually Transmitted Diseases. Clin Colon Rectal Surg. 2004 November; 17(4): 209–214.

30 Dorward DW, Fischer ER, Brooks DM. Invasion and cytopathic killing of human lymphocytes by spirochetes causing Lyme disease. *Clinical Infectious Diseases* 1997; 25 (S1): 2–8.

31 Dorward DW, Larson RS. Murine model for lymphocytic tropism by Borrelia burgdorferi. *Infection and Immunity* 2001; 69(3): 1428–32.

32 Coburn J, Fischer JR, Leong JM. Solving a sticky problem: new genetic approaches to host cell adhesion by the Lyme disease spirochete. *Molecular Microbiology* 2005; 57(5): 1182–95.

33 Fumarola D, Cedola MC, Guanti G, Matsuura A, Uede T, Jirillo E. Adherence of Lyme disease spirochetes to rat lymphocytes. *Zentralbl Bakteriol Mikrobiol Hyg A.* 1986; 263(1-2): 146-50.

34 Hsi Liu DSM, Steiner BM, Schnell RF. In Vivo Immunotherapy of Treponemal Infection by Depletion of CD4 T Cells. *Journal of Spirochetal and Tick-borne Diseases* 2002; 9: 3-10.

35 Cruz AR, Ramirez LG, Zuluaga AV, et al. Immune Evasion and Recognition of the Syphilis Spirochete in Blood and Skin of Secondary Syphilis Patients: Two Immunologically Distinct Compartments. PLoS Negl Trop Dis. 2012;6(7):e1717.

36 Schlesinger PA, Duray PH, Burke BA, Steere AC, Stillman MT. Maternal-fetal transmission of the Lyme disease spirochete, Borrelia burgdorferi. Ann Intern Med. 1985 Jul;103(1):67-8.

37 Oliver J. SYPHILITIC DISEASE OF THE THYMUS IN INFANTS AND THE MODE OF ORIGIN OF THE DUBOIS ABSCESSES. Am J Dis Child. 1917;13(2):158-166.

38 Hütter G, Nowak D, Mossner M, et al. Long-term control of HIV by CCR5 Delta32/Delta32 stem-cell transplantation. N Engl J Med. 2009 Feb 12;360(7):692-8.

39 Sellatil TJ, Wilkinson DA, Sheffield JS, Koup RA, Radolf JD, Norgard MV. Virulent Treponema pallidum, Lipoprotein, and Synthetic Lipopeptides Induce CCR5 on Human Monocytes and Enhance Their Susceptibility to Infection by Human Immunodeficiency Virus Type 1. *J Infect Dis.* 2000; 181 (1): 283–293.

40 Zagzag D. The Role of SDF1-∝ and CXCR4 In the Pathogenesis of Lyme Disease of the Central And Peripheral Nervous System. *Lyme Neuroborreliosis Research Program.* Online at http://www.lymeneuroborreliosisprogram.org/html/current-research/current-studies/study-no-2.html, accessed on December 18, 2013.

41 Salazar JC, Cruz AR, Pope CD, et al. Treponema pallidum elicits innate and adaptive cellular immune responses in skin and blood during secondary syphilis: a flow-cytometric analysis. *J Infect Dis.* 2007;195 (6): 879–87.

42 Monteiro de Almeida S, Bhatt A, Riggs PK, et al. Cerebrospinal fluid human immunodeficiency virus viral load in patients with neurosyphilis. J Neurovirol. 2010 February; 16(1): 6–12.

43 Salazar JC, et al. Lipoprotein-Dependent and -Independent Immune Responses to Spirochetal Infection. Clin Diagn Lab Immunol. 2005; 12 (8): 949–958.

44 Ormsby CE, Gupta DS, Tandon R, et al. Human Endogenous Retrovirus Expression Is Inversely Associated with Chronic Immune Activation in HIV-1 Infection. PLoS One. 2012; 7(8): e41021.

45 Norgard MV, Arndt LL, Akins DR Curetty LL, Harrich DA, Radolf JD. Activation of human monocytic cells by Treponema pallidum and Borrelia burgdorferi lipoproteins and synthetic lipopeptides proceeds via a pathway distinct from that of lipopolysaccharide but involves the transcriptional activator NF-kappa B. *Infect. Immun.* 1996; 64 (9): 3845–3852.

46 Hashemi FB, Ghassemi M, Roebuck KA, Spear GT. Activation of Human Immunodeficiency Virus Type 1 Expression by Gardnerella vaginalis. *J Infect Dis.* 1999; 179 (4): 924–930.

47 Zajac V, Stevurkova V, Matelova L, Ujhazy E. Detection of HIV-1 sequences in intestinal bacteria of HIV/AIDS patients. *Neuro Endocrinol Lett.* 2007; 28(5): 591-5.

48 Sadiq ST, McSorley J, Copas AJ, et al. The effects of early syphilis on CD4 counts and HIV-1 RNA viral loads in blood and semen. *Sex Transm Infect* 2005; 81: 380–385.

49 Jarzebowski W, Caumes E, Dupin N, et al. Effect of early syphilis infection on plasma viral load and CD4 cell count in human immunodeficiency virus-infected men: results from the FHDH-ANRS CO4 cohort. *Arch Intern Med.* 2012; 172 (16): 1237–43.

50 Chandler FW, McClure HM, Campbell WG, Watts JC. Pulmonary pneumocystosis in nonhuman primates. Archives of Pathology & Laboratory Medicine 1976; 100(3):163-167.

51 Hsu PL, Qin M, Norris SJ, and Sell S. Isolation and characterization of recombinant Escherichia coli clones secreting a 24-kilodalton antigen of Treponema pallidum. Infect Immun. 1988 May; 56(5): 1135–1143.

52 Poltavchenko AG, Rybakov AN, Nadtochiĭ ON. Dynamics of humoral immune response to Treponema pallidum proteins p17 and p41 at early stages of syphilis. Zh Mikrobiol Epidemiol Immunobiol. 2004 May-Jun;(3):52-7.

53 Magnarelli LA, Fikrig E, Padula SJ, Anderson JF, Flavell RA. Use of recombinant antigens of Borrelia burgdorferi in serologic tests for diagnosis of lyme borreliosis. J Clin Microbiol. 1996 Feb;34(2):237-40.

54 Pinter A, Honnen WJ, Tilley SA, et al. Oligomeric Structure of gp4l, the Transmembrane Protein of Human Immunodeficiency Virus Type 1. JOURNAL OF VIROLOGY 1989; 63(6): 2674-2679.

55 Tseng CK, Hughes MA, Hsu PL, Mahoney S, Duvic M, Sell S. Syphilis superinfection activates expression of human immunodeficiency virus I in latently infected rabbits. Am J Pathol. 1991 May;138(5):1149-64.

56 Theus SA, Harrich DA, Gaynor R, Radolf JD, Norgard MV. Treponema pallidum, Lipoproteins, and Synthetic Lipoprotein Analogues Induce Human Immunodeficiency Virus Type 1 Gene Expression in Monocytes via NF-κB Activation. J Infect Dis. 1998; 177 (4): 941–950.

57 Eriksson S, Graf EH, Dahl V, et al. Comparative analysis of measures of viral reservoirs in HIV-1 eradication studies. PLoS Pathog. 2013 Feb;9(2):e1003174.

58 Ryan FP. Viruses as symbionts. Symbiosis 2007; 44 (1): 11–21.

59 Brorson O, Brorson SH, Scythes J, MacAllister J, Wier A, Margulis L. Destruction of spirochete Borrelia burgdorferi round-body propagules (RBs) by the antibiotic Tigecycline. *Proc Natl Acad Sci U S A*. 2009; 106(44): 18656–18661.

60 Margulis L, Maniotis A, MacAllister J, et al. Spirochete round bodies, Syphilis, Lyme disease & AIDS: Resurgence of "the great imitator"? *Symbiosis* 2009; 47 (1): 51–58.

61 Salado-Rasmussen K, Katzenstein TL, Gerstoft J, et al. Risk of HIV or second syphilis infection in Danish men with newly acquired syphilis in the period 2000–2010. *Sex Transm Infect.* 2013; 89 (5): 372-6.

62 Funnyé AS, Akhtar AJ. Syphilis and human immunodeficiency virus co-infection. J Natl Med Assoc. 2003 May; 95(5): 363–382. conifection 60 to 90% in MSM, false-negative

63 Lynn WA, Lightman S. Syphilis and HIV: a dangerous combination. Lancet Infect Dis. 2004 Jul;4(7):456-66.

64 Kark SL. The social pathology of syphilis in Africans. Int J Epidemiol. 2003 Apr;32(2):181-6.

65 Lafeuillade A, Quilichini R, Benderitter R, Delbeke E, Dhiver C, Gastaut JA. Intestinal spirochaetosis in HIV infected homosexual men. *Postgrad Med J.* 1990; 66 (773): 253–254.

66 Law CL, Grierson JM, Stevens SM. Rectal spirochaetosis in homosexual men: the association with sexual practices, HIV infection and enteric flora. *Genitourin Med.* 1994; 70(1): 26–9.

67 Cooper C, Cotton DW, Hudson MJ, Kirkham N, Wilmott FE. Rectal spirochaetosis in homosexual men: characterisation of the organism and pathophysiology. *Genitourin Med.* 1986; 62 (1): 47–52.

68 Tsinganou E, Gebbers JO. Human intestinal spirochetosis – a review. *Ger Med Sci.* 2010; 8:Doc01

69 Hébert-Schuster M, Borderie D, Grange PA, et al. Oxidative stress markers are increased since early stages of infection in syphilitic patients. Arch Dermatol Res. 2012 Nov;304(9):689-97.

70 Seyfried TN, Shelton LM. Cancer as a metabolic disease. Nutr Metab (Lond). 2010 Jan 27;7:7

71 Jaeger H, Geiser D. Sur la sarcomatose de Kaposi et son traitement par la pénicilline. Dermatologica 1954; 108:366–373

72 Fayolle J et al. La Penicilline dans le Traitement de I'Angiosarcomatose de Kaposi. Lyon Medical 1980; 244:(17): 277-281.

73 Halperin DT. Heterosexual anal intercourse: prevalence, cultural factors, and HIV infection and other health risks, Part I. AIDS Patient Care STDS. 1999 Dec;13(12):717-30.

74 Scythes JB, Jones CM. Syphilis in the AIDS era: diagnostic dilemma and therapeutic challenge. *Acta Microbiologica et Immunologica Hungarica* 2013; 60 (2): 93–116.

75 Fitzgerald F. The great imitator, syphilis. West J Med. 1981 May;134(5):424-32. symptoms, 1 to 9 unreported, not conquered

76 Michalek AM, Mahoney MC, McLaughlin CC, Murphy D, Metzger BB. Historical and contemporary correlates of syphilis and cancer. *Int J Epidemiol.* 1994; 23 (2): 381–5.

77 Kaposi M. Idiopathisches multiples Pigmentsarkom der Haut. Archiv für Dermatologie und Syphilis 1872; 4(2): 265-273.

78 Farhi DC, Wells SJ, Siegel RJ. Syphilitic lymphadenopathy. Histology and human immunodeficiency virus status. Am J Clin Pathol. 1999 Sep;112(3):330-4.

79 Goffinet DR, Hoyt C, Eltringham JR. Secondary syphilis misdiagnosed as a lymphoma. Calif Med. 1970 May; 112(5): 22–23.

80 MONTGOMERY DW, CULVER GD. LUETIC LYMPHOMA IN LATE SYPHILIS. JAMA. 1910;LIV(8):605-607.

81 Goffinet DR, Hoyt C, Eltringham JR. Secondary syphilis misdiagnosed as a lymphoma. Calif Med. 1970 May; 112(5): 22–23.

82 Acharya V, Varghese GK, Roy A. Secondary syphilis mimicking cutaneous lymphoma. J Indian Med Assoc. 2011 Mar;109(3):196-7.

83 Bramkamp AL. ASSOCIATED SYPHILIS AND TUBERCULOSIS. Cal State J Med. 1923 February; 21(2): 52–55.

84 Goldblatt S. RELATION BETWEEN SYPHILIS AND TUBERCULOSIS IN THE NEGRO. Arch Derm Syphilol. 1939;40(5):792-802.

85 Collart P, Borel LJ, Durel P. Significance of Spiral Organisms Found, after Treatment, in Late Human and Experimental Syphilis. Br J Vener Dis. 1964 June; 40(2): 81–89.

86 Ovcinnikov NM, Delektorskij VV. Effect of crystalline penicillin and bicillin-1 on experimental syphilis in the rabbit. Electron microscope study. Br J Vener Dis. 1972 October; 48(5): 327–341.

87 Ovcinnikov NM, Korbut SE, Bednova VN, Timcenko GF, Milonova TI. Long-term results of penicillin treatment of early and late forms of syphilis in the rabbit. Br J Vener Dis. 1973 October; 49(5): 413–419.

88 Hodzic E, Feng S, Holden K, Freet K, Barthold SW. Persistence of Borrelia burgdorferi Following Antibiotic Treatment in Mice. *Antimicro Agents Chemother* 2008; 52 (5): 1728–1736.

89 Hunfeld KP, Ruzic-Sabljic E, Norris DE, Kraiczy P, Strle F. In Vitro Susceptibility Testing of Borrelia burgdorferi Sensu Lato Isolates Cultured from Patients with Erythema Migrans before and after Antimicrobial Chemotherapy. *Antimicro Agents Chemother* 2005; 49 (4): 1294–1301.

90 Chang YF, Ku YW, Chang CF, et al. Antibiotic treatment of experimentally Borrelia burgdorferi-infected ponies. *Vet Microbio* 2005; 107 (3-4): 285–294.

91 Fried MD, Pietrucha D, Madigan G, Bal A. Borrelia burgdorferi Persists in the Gastrointestinal Tract of Children and Adolescents with Lyme Disease. *Journal of Spirochetal and Tick-borne Diseases* 2002; 9: 11–15.

92 Ovcinnikov NM, Delektorskij VV. Treponema pallidum in nerve fibres. Br J Vener Dis. 1975 February; 51(1): 10–18.

93 Lukehart SA, Hook EW 3rd, Baker-Zander SA, et al. Invasion of the central nervous system by Treponema pallidum: implications for diagnosis and treatment. Ann Intern Med. 1988 Dec 1;109(11):855-62.

94 Ho EL, Lukehart SA. Syphilis: using modern approaches to understand an old disease. J Clin Invest. 2011 December 1; 121(12): 4584–4592.

95 Sykes JA, Miller JN. Intracellular Location of Treponema pallidum (Nichols Strain) in the Rabbit Testis. Infect Immun. 1971 September; 4(3): 307–314.

96 Lauderdale V, Goldman JN. Serial ultrathin sectioning demonstrating the intracellularity of T. Pallidum. An electron microscopic study. Br J Vener Dis. 1972 April; 48(2): 87–96.

97 Sykes JA, Miller JN, Kalan AJ. Treponema pallidum within cells of a primary chancre from a human female. Br J Vener Dis. 1974 February; 50(1): 40–44.

98 Ovcinnikov NM, Delektorskij VV. Current concepts of the morphology and biology of Treponema pallidum based on electron microscopy. Br J Vener Dis. 1971 October; 47(5): 315–328.

99 Umemoto T, Namikawa I, Yoshii Z, Konishi H. An internal view of the spherical body of Treponema macrodentium as revealed by scanning electron microscopy. Microbiol Immunol. 1982;26(3):191-8.

100 Carlson JA, Dabiri G, Cribier B, Sell S. The immunopathobiology of syphilis: the manifestations and course of syphilis are determined by the level of delayed-type hypersensitivity. Am J Dermatopathol. 2011 Jul;33(5):433-60.

101 Hicks CB, Benson PM, Lupton GP, Tramont EC. Seronegative secondary syphilis in a patient infected with the human immunodeficiency virus (HIV) with Kaposi sarcoma. A diagnostic dilemma. Ann Intern Med. 1987 Oct;107(4):492-5.

102 Haas JS, Bolan G, Larsen SA, Clement MJ, Bacchetti P, Moss AR. Sensitivity of treponemal tests for detecting prior treated syphilis during human immunodeficiency virus infection. J Infect Dis. 1990 Oct;162(4):862-6.

103 Janier M, Chastang C, Spindler E, et al. A prospective study of the influence of HIV status on the seroreversion of serological tests for syphilis. Dermatology. 1999;198(4):362-9.

104 Johnson PD, Graves SR, Stewart L, Warren R, Dwyer B, Lucas CR. Specific syphilis serological tests may become negative in HIV infection. AIDS. 1991 Apr;5(4):419-23.

105 Erbelding EJ, Vlahov D, Nelson KE, et al. Syphilis serology in human immunodeficiency virus infection: evidence for false-negative fluorescent treponemal testing. J Infect Dis. 1997 Nov;176(5):1397-400.

106 Telzak EE, Greenberg MS, Harrison J, Stoneburner RL, Schultz S. Syphilis treatment response in HIV-infected individuals. AIDS. 1991 May;5(5):591-5.

107 Ghanem KG, Erbelding EJ, Wiener ZS, Rompalo AM. Serological response to syphilis treatment in HIV-positive and HIV-negative patients attending sexually transmitted diseases clinics. Sex Transm Infect. 2007 Apr;83(2):97-101.

108 Radolf JD, Desrosiers DC. Treponema pallidum, the Stealth Pathogen, Doth Change, But How? Mol Microbiol. 2009 June; 72(5): 1081–1086.

109 Cox DL, Chang P, McDowall AW, Radolf JD. The outer membrane, not a coat of host proteins, limits antigenicity of virulent Treponema pallidum. Infect Immun. 1992 Mar;60(3):1076-83.

110 Izard J, Renken C, Hsieh CE, et al. Cryo-electron tomography elucidates the molecular architecture of Treponema pallidum, the syphilis spirochete. J Bacteriol. 2009 Dec;191(24):7566-80.

111 Liu J, Howell JK, Bradley SD, Zheng Y, Zhou ZH, Norris SJ. Cellular architecture of Treponema pallidum: novel flagellum, periplasmic cone, and cell envelope as revealed by cryo electron tomography. J Mol Biol. 2010 Nov 5;403(4):546-61.

112 Radolf JD. Role of outer membrane architecture in immune evasion by Treponema pallidum and Borrelia burgdorferi. Trends Microbiol. 1994 Sep;2(9):307-11.

113 Radolf JD. Treponema pallidum and the quest for outer membrane proteins. Mol Microbiol. 1995 Jun;16(6):1067-73.

114 Barbour AG, Dai Q, Restrepo BI, Stoenner HG, Frank SA. Pathogen escape from host immunity by a genome program for antigenic variation. Proc Natl Acad Sci U S A. 2006 Nov 28;103(48):18290-5.

115 Giacani L, Molini BJ, Kim EY, et al. Antigenic variation in Treponema pallidum: TprK sequence diversity accumulates in response to immune pressure during experimental syphilis. J Immunol. 2010 Apr 1;184(7):3822-9.

116 Thompson JJ, Mangi RJ, Lee R, Dwyer JM. Immunoregulatory properties of serum from patients with different stages of syphilis. Br J Vener Dis. 1980 August; 56(4): 210–217.

117 Pavia CS, Folds JD, Baseman JB. Cell-mediated immunity during syphilis. A review. Br J Vener Dis. 1978 June; 54(3): 144–150.

118 Seña AC, White BL, Sparling PF. Novel Treponema pallidum serologic tests: a paradigm shift in syphilis screening for the 21st century. *Clin Infect Dis.* 2010; 51 (6): 700–8.

119 Grange PA, Gressier L, Dion PL, et al. Evaluation of a PCR test for detection of treponema pallidum in swabs and blood. J Clin Microbiol. 2012 Mar;50(3):546-52.

120 Shields M, Guy RJ, Jeoffreys NJ, Finlayson RJ, Donovan B. A longitudinal evaluation of Treponema pallidum PCR testing in early syphilis. BMC Infect Dis. 2012 Dec 17;12:353.

121 Boeck W. On syphilization. The Dublin Quarterly Journal of Medical Science February 1, 1857, Volume 23, Issue 1, pp 77-87.

122 Stillians AW. SYPHILIZATIONAN EPISODE IN THE EVOLUTION OF SYPHILOLOGY. Arch Derm Syphilol. 1938;37(2):272-278.

123 Sherwood J. Syphilization: Human Experimentation in the Search for a Syphilis Vaccine in the Nineteenth Century. J Hist Med Allied Sci (1999) 54 (3): 364-386.

124 Buchbinder SP, Katz MH, Hessol NA, O'Malley PM, Holmberg SD. Long-term HIV-1 infection without immunologic progression. AIDS 1994; 8 (8): 1123–8.

125 Ghanem KG, Moore RD, Rompalo AM, Erbelding EJ, Zenilman JM, Gebo KA. Antiretroviral Therapy Is Associated with Reduced Serologic Failure Rates for Syphilis among HIV-Infected Patients. Clinical Infectious Diseases 2008; 47 (2): 258–265.

126 Modjarrad K, Vermund SH. Effect of treating co-infections on HIV-1 viral load: a systematic review. Lancet Infect Dis. 2010 Jul;10(7):455-63.

127 Ladinsky MS et al. Electron Tomography of HIV-1 Infection in Gut-Associated Lymphoid Tissue. PLoS Pathog 2014; 10(1): e1003899. doi:10.1371/journal.ppat.1003899

www.ingramcontent.com/pod-product-compliance
Lightning Source LLC
Chambersburg PA
CBHW071808170526
45167CB00003B/1221